A New Mediterranean Diet Cookbook For Beginners

Simple Meal Plan and 28- day Recipes For Weight Loss Management

Allen A. Cary

CONTENTS

Introduction

Mediterranean Diet Cookbook: An Introduction

The principles of the Mediterranean diet are the focus of an extensive manual and recipe collection referred to as The Mediterranean Diet Cookbook. The traditional eating patterns of residents of Mediterranean Sea-bordering nations, which include Greece, Italy, Spain, and Morocco, are the inspiration for this diet.

Due to its many health advantages and emphasis on fresh, whole foods, the Mediterranean diet has attracted a lot of attention and popularity. It is well known for aiding heart health, managing weight, and general wellbeing. The diet emphasises eating foods high in nutrients, such as fruits, vegetables, whole grains, legumes, nuts, seeds, and olive oil. Moderate amounts of seafood, poultry, dairy products, and red wine are also included.

A variety of meals can be found in The Mediterranean Diet Cookbook.

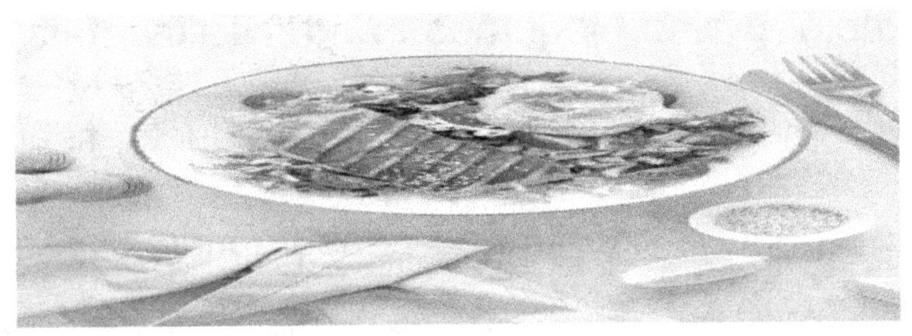

Chapter 1: The Basics of the Mediterranean Diet

The Mediterranean Diet Pyramid: A Visual Guide

The Mediterranean diet pyramid is a nutritional guideline that represents the traditional dietary pattern followed by people in the Mediterranean region. It emphasises a high consumption of fruits, vegetables, whole grains, legumes, and healthy fats, with moderate intake of dairy products, fish, and poultry, and limited consumption of red meat and sweets. Here is a breakdown of the Mediterranean diet pyramid from the base to the top:

Physical activity: The pyramid emphasises the importance of regular physical activity, such as walking, gardening, or participating in sports.

Water: Water is the main beverage recommended for hydration. It suggests drinking plenty of water throughout the day.

Olive oil: Olive oil is a primary source of fat in the Mediterranean diet. It is rich in monounsaturated fats and antioxidants and is used as the primary cooking oil and dressing.

Fruits, vegetables, legumes, and nuts: The pyramid encourages a high consumption of these foods, which are rich in vitamins, minerals, fibre, and antioxidants. They should be included in every meal and snack.

Whole grains and cereals: This category includes whole grain bread, pasta, rice, and other cereals. Whole grains are a good source of fibre and nutrients and should be consumed in moderation.

Fish, poultry, and eggs: Fish and seafood, such as salmon, sardines, and shrimp, are recommended at least twice a week. Poultry, such as chicken and turkey, is consumed in moderation, while eggs are included but limited to a few servings per week.

Dairy products: Moderate amounts of dairy products like yoghurt and cheese are part of the Mediterranean diet. However, it is recommended to choose low-fat or skim options.

Red meat and sweets: Red meat and sweets, including processed meats, should be consumed in limited amounts and considered occasional treats rather than regular components of the diet.

The Mediterranean diet pyramid promotes a balanced and varied approach to eating, with an emphasis on whole, minimally processed foods. It has been associated with numerous health benefits, including reduced risk of heart disease, stroke, and certain types of cancer, as well as improved weight management and overall well-being.

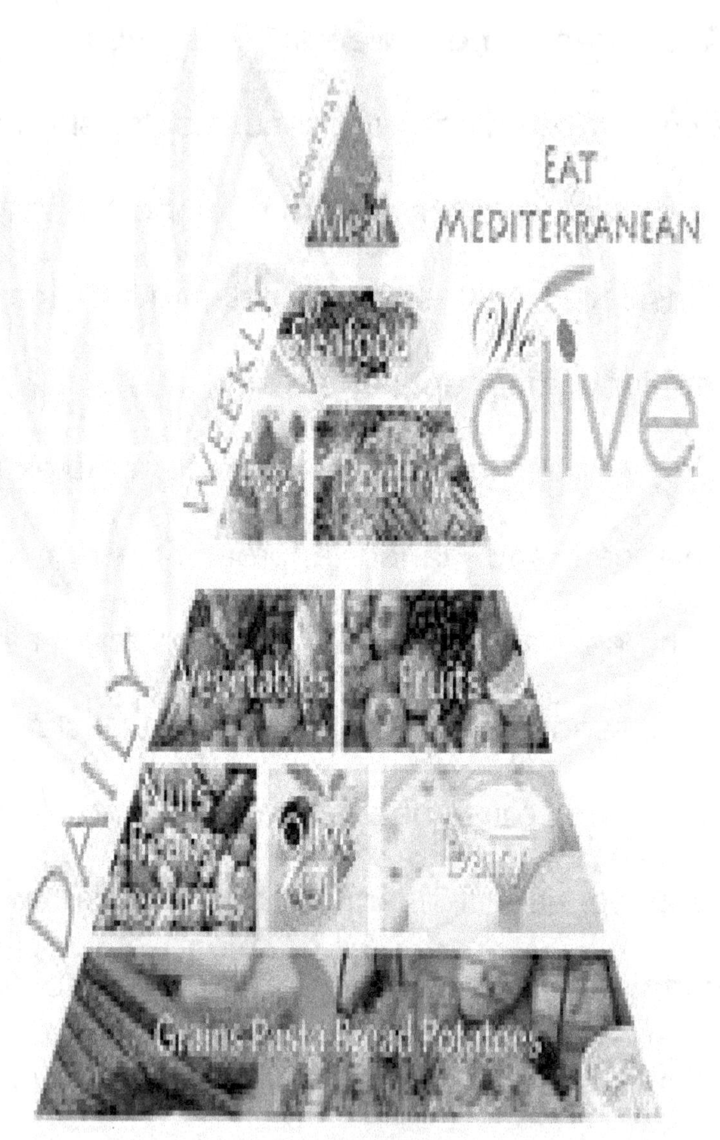

EAT
MEDITERRANEAN
We olive
Monthly
Meat
WEEKLY
Seafood
Eggs
Poultry
Vegetables
Fruits
Nuts
Beans
Legumes
Olive Oil
Dairy
DAILY
Grains Pasta Bread Potatoes

Staples of the Mediterranean Pantry

The Mediterranean pantry is known for its abundance of fresh and flavorful ingredients. Here are some staples commonly found in a Mediterranean pantry:

I

Olive Oil: This is a fundamental ingredient in Mediterranean cuisine. Extra virgin olive oil is used for cooking, dressing salads, and adding flavour to various dishes.

Tomatoes: Whether fresh or canned, tomatoes are a versatile ingredient used in numerous Mediterranean recipes, such as pasta sauces, stews, and salads.

Garlic: Known for its strong aroma and taste, garlic is a key ingredient in Mediterranean cooking. It is used to add flavour to sauces, marinades, roasted vegetables, and more.

Herbs and spices: Mediterranean cuisine relies heavily on herbs and spices to enhance the flavours of dishes. Common options include oregano, basil, thyme, rosemary, parsley, cumin, coriander, and paprika.

Olives: A variety of olives, both green and black, are widely used in Mediterranean cooking. They can be enjoyed as a snack, incorporated into salads, or used as a garnish for various dishes.

Canned Fish: Tinned fish, such as tuna, sardines, and anchovies, are frequently used in Mediterranean recipes. They are often added to salads, pasta dishes, and spreads like tapenade.

Beans and Legumes: Chickpeas, lentils, and white beans are commonly found in Mediterranean recipes. They are used in soups, stews, salads, and dips like hummus.

Pasta and Grains: Mediterranean cuisine includes a variety of pasta shapes, such as spaghetti, penne, and orzo. Grains like couscous, bulgur, and rice are also commonly used.

Nuts and Seeds: Almonds, walnuts, pine nuts, and sesame seeds are frequently used in Mediterranean cooking. They are added to salads, desserts, and various dishes for texture and flavour.

Citrus Fruits: Lemons, oranges, and other citrus fruits are prevalent in Mediterranean cuisine. They are used for their juice and zest and as a refreshing addition to salads and marinades. These are just a few examples of the staples you might find in a Mediterranean pantry. The region's cuisine is diverse, so the specific ingredients may vary depending on the country and local traditions within the Mediterranean region.

Essential Cooking Techniques and Tools

When it comes to cooking, there are several essential techniques and tools that every home cook should know and have in their kitchen. **Here are some of the Cooking Techniques:**

Sautéing: This technique involves cooking food quickly in a small amount of oil or fat over high heat. It's commonly used for browning vegetables, searing meat, and creating stir-fries.

Roasting: Roasting is a dry-heat cooking method that involves cooking food in the oven at a high temperature. It's great for cooking meat, poultry, and vegetables, resulting in delicious caramelization and browning.

Grilling: Grilling involves cooking food over direct heat, usually on a grill or barbecue. It's a popular technique for cooking meat, seafood, and vegetables, imparting a smoky flavour.

Boiling: Boiling is the process of cooking food in boiling water or another liquid. It's commonly used for pasta, rice, vegetables, and making stocks and soups.

Braising: Braising involves browning meat or vegetables and then cooking them slowly in a covered pot with a small amount of liquid. It's a great technique for tenderising tough cuts of meat and developing rich flavours.

Chef's Knife: A good-quality chef's knife is essential for chopping, slicing, and dicing ingredients. Look for a knife with a sharp, sturdy blade and a comfortable handle.

Cutting Board: A durable cutting board provides a safe and hygienic surface for chopping and preparing food. Opt for one made of wood or plastic that is large enough to accommodate your ingredients.

Mixing Bowls: Having a set of mixing bowls in various sizes is useful for preparing and combining ingredients. Stainless steel or glass bowls are the most common options.

Pots and Pans: Invest in a set of high-quality pots and pans with different sizes and types, such as a saucepan, sauté pan, and stockpot. Choose materials that distribute heat evenly, like stainless steel or cast iron.

Wooden Spoon: A wooden spoon is versatile and won't scratch your cookware. It's useful for stirring, mixing, and scraping the bottom of pans.

Tongs: Tongs are great for flipping meat, tossing salads, and handling hot food. Look for tongs with long handles and a good grip.

Whisk: Whisks are essential for beating eggs, mixing sauces, and incorporating air into batters. Choose one with thin wires and a comfortable handle.

Measuring Cups and Spoons: Accurate measurements are crucial in cooking, so having a set of measuring cups and spoons is essential for both dry and liquid ingredients.

Oven Mitts or Potholders: These protect your hands from hot cookware and oven temperatures. Look for heat-resistant materials that provide a good grip.

Kitchen Timer: A kitchen timer helps you keep track of cooking times and prevents overcooking or burning. You can use a physical timer or use the timer function on your phone or oven.

These are just a few of the many cooking techniques and tools available, but they cover the basics for most home cooking needs. As you explore and expand your culinary skills, you may discover more techniques and tools that suit your cooking

style and preferences.

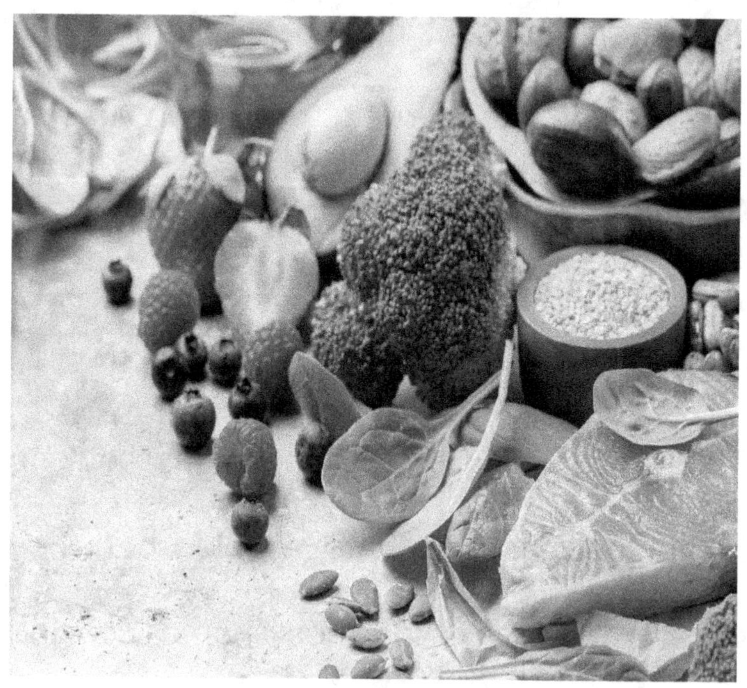

Classic Greek Yogurt Parfait

Greek yoghourt parfait is a delicious and nutritious breakfast or snack option that combines layers of Greek yoghurt, fresh fruits, and granola. It's a versatile dish that allows for customization based on personal preferences and dietary needs. Here's a simple recipe to make a Greek yoghourt parfait:

Ingredients:

1 cup of Greek yoghourt

1 cup mixed fresh berries (such as strawberries, blueberries, and raspberries)

1/2 cup granola

1 tablespoon honey (optional, for added sweetness)

Fresh mint leaves for garnish (optional)

Instructions:

Start by selecting a clear glass or bowl to create beautiful layers in your parfait.

Begin with a layer of Greek yoghurt at the bottom of the glass. Use about 1/4 cup of yoghurt.

Add a layer of mixed fresh berries on top of the yoghurt. You can use any combination of berries you like. Sprinkle a layer of granola over the berries. This adds a crunchy texture to the parfait. Repeat the layers by adding another layer of Greek yoghurt, berries, and granola. Drizzle a tablespoon of honey over the top layer for extra sweetness, if desired.

Garnish with fresh mint leaves for a touch of freshness and presentation. Serve immediately, and enjoy. You can customise your Greek yoghourt parfait by adding different fruits, such as sliced bananas or peaches, or incorporating additional toppings like nuts, coconut flakes, or chia seeds. It's a versatile recipe that allows you to experiment and create your own delicious combinations.

Feta and Spinach Omelette

Feta and spinach omelette is a delicious and nutritious dish that combines the creaminess of feta cheese with the freshness of spinach. It's a popular choice for a healthy breakfast or brunch. Here's a simple recipe to make a feta and spinach omelette:

Ingredients:

3 large eggs

1 cup fresh spinach leaves, chopped

1/4 cup crumbled feta cheese

Salt and pepper to taste; 1 tablespoon olive oil or butter

Instructions:

In a bowl, crack the eggs and whisk them until well beaten. Season with salt and pepper according to your taste.

Heat the olive oil or butter in a non-stick skillet over medium heat.

Add the chopped spinach to the skillet and sauté for about 2 minutes until wilted.

Pour the beaten eggs into the skillet, ensuring that the spinach is evenly distributed.

Allow the eggs to cook undisturbed for a minute or two until the edges start to set.

Sprinkle the crumbled feta cheese evenly over the omelette.

Using a spatula, gently fold the omelette in half, covering the filling.

Cook for another minute, or until the eggs are fully cooked and the cheese is melted.

Carefully slide the omelette onto a plate and serve hot.

You can also customise this recipe by adding other ingredients like diced tomatoes, sliced mushrooms, or diced onions for extra flavour. Enjoy your feta and spinach omelette!

Olive Oil Pancakes with Citrus Compote

pancakes with Compote compote are a delicious and flavorful twist on traditional pancakes. Live-edition of olive oil in the batter gives the pancakes a rich and slightly savoury taste, while the citrus compote adds a tangy and refreshing element. Here's a recipe to help you make these delightful pancakes:

Ingredients for Olive Oil Pancakes:

1 1/2 cups all-pancakes: loPancakes: spoons granulated flour ar

1 tablespoons of baking popsugar /2 teaspoon baking soda

1/4 teaspoon salt

1 cup of buttermilk

1/2 cup milk

2 large eggs

3 tablespoons extra virgin olive oil

1 teaspoon of vanilla extract

Ingredients for Citrus Compote:

2 oranges

2 lemons

2 tablespoons of honey

1/4 cup of water

Zest of 1 orange Zest of 1 lemon

Instructions:

In a large mixing bowl, whisk together the flour, sugar, baking powder, baking soda, and salt.

In a separate bowl, combine the buttermilk, milk, eggs, olive oil, and vanilla extract. Whisk until well combined.

Pour the wet ingredients into the dry ingredients and gently stir until just combined. Be careful not to overmix; a few lumps are okay.

Preheat a griddle or non-stick skillet over medium heat. Lightly grease the surface with olive oil or cooking spray.

Pour about 1/4 cup of batter onto the griddle for each pancake. Cook until bubbles form on the surface, then flip and cook for another 1-2 minutes, or until golden brown.

Transfer the cooked pancakes to a plate and cover with a clean kitchen towel to keep them warm while you make the citrus compote.

Juice one orange and one lemon, and set the juice aside.

Peel the remaining orange and lemon, removing as much of the pith as possible. Segment the fruits by cutting between the membranes to remove the individual citrus sections. Set aside.

In a small saucepan, combine the honey, water, and citrus juice. Heat over medium heat until the mixture comes to a simmer.

Add the orange and lemon segments to the saucepan along with the orange and lemon zest. Stir gently to coat the segments with the liquid.

Cook the compote for about 5-7 minutes, stirring occasionally, until the citrus segments are softened and the liquid has thickened slightly.

Remove the compote from the heat and let it cool slightly.

To serve, stack the olive oil pancakes on a plate and spoon the citrus compote on top. You can garnish with additional zest or a drizzle of honey if desired. Enjoy your delicious olive oil pancakes with citrus compote!

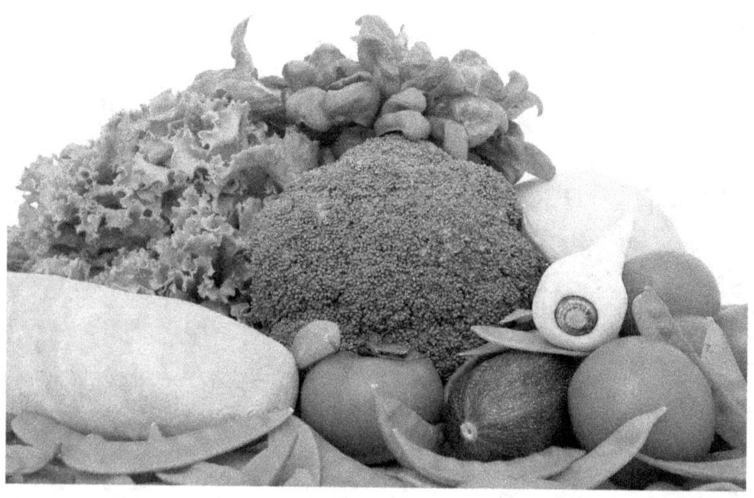

Roasted Red Pepper Hummus

Roasted Red Pepper Hummus is a delicious and healthy dip made from chickpeas, roasted red peppers, tahini (sesame seed paste), garlic, lemon juice, and various spices. It's a popular Middle Eastern dish that has gained worldwide popularity for its flavorful and creamy texture.

Here's a simple recipe to make roasted red pepper hummus:

Ingredients:

- 1 can (15 ounces) chickpeas (garbanzo beans), drained and rinsed

- 1 large roasted red pepper (you can roast it yourself or use jarred roasted red peppers)

- 3 tablespoons tahini, 2 cloves garlic, minced

- 2 tablespoons of lemon juice

- 2 tablespoons of olive oil

- 1/2 teaspoon ground cumin

- 1/2 teaspoon paprika

- Salt and pepper to taste

Instructions:

In a food processor or blender, combine the chickpeas, roasted red pepper, tahini, garlic, lemon juice, olive oil, cumin, paprika, salt, and pepper.

Blend the mixture until smooth and creamy. If needed, you can add a little water to thin it out to your desired consistency.

Taste the hummus and adjust the seasoning if necessary. You can add more lemon juice, salt, or any other spices according to your preference.

Once the hummus reaches your desired taste and consistency, transfer it to a serving bowl. You can garnish the hummus with a drizzle of olive oil, a sprinkle of paprika, and some chopped fresh herbs like parsley or cilantro.

Serve the roasted red pepper hummus with pita bread, tortilla chips, and fresh vegetables, or use it as a spread for sandwiches and wraps. Enjoy your homemade roasted red pepper hummus!

Marinated Olives and Feta Skewer

Marinated Olives and Feta Skewers are a delicious and flavorful appetiser or snack that combines the tanginess of marinated olives with the creaminess of feta cheese. Here's a simple recipe to make these skewers:

Ingredients:

- 1 cup mixed olives (such as Kalamata, green, or black olives)

- 1 cup feta cheese, cut into bite-sized cubes

- 2 tablespoons of olive oil

- 1 tablespoon of lemon juice

- 1 clove of garlic, minced

- 1 teaspoon dried oregano

- Freshly ground black pepper, to taste

- Skewers or toothpicks

Instructions:

In a bowl, combine the olive oil, lemon juice, minced garlic, dried oregano, and black pepper. Whisk the ingredients together to create the marinade.

Add the olives to the marinade and toss them until they are well coated. Allow the olives to marinate for at least 30 minutes to absorb the flavours. You can refrigerate them if you marinate them for a longer time.

Preheat your grill or broiler to medium-high heat.

Thread the marinated olives and feta cheese cubes onto skewers or toothpicks, alternating between the two.

Place the skewers on the grill or under the broiler and cook for about 2–3 minutes per side, or until the feta cheese starts to soften and slightly melt.

Remove the skewers from the heat and let them cool slightly before serving.

Serve the marinated olives and feta skewers as an appetiser or snack. They can be enjoyed warm or at room temperature.

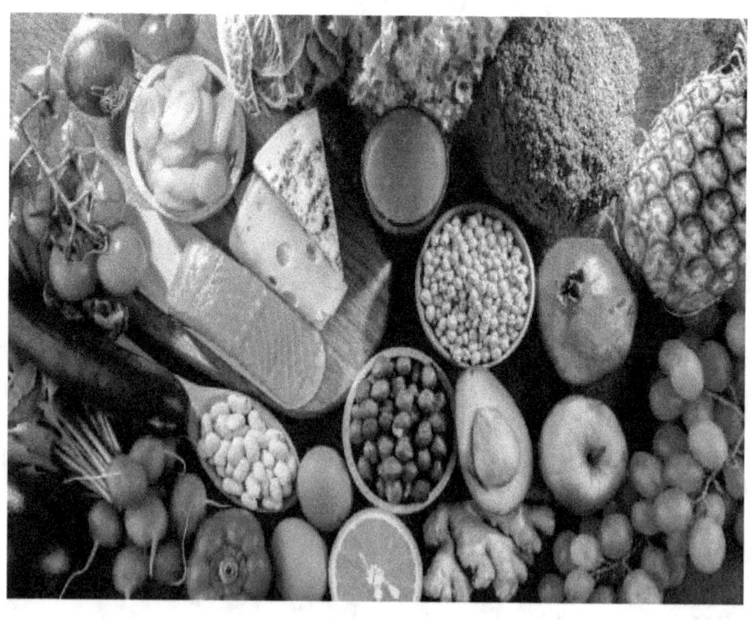

Greek Salad with Grilled Halloumi

Greek Salad with Grilled Halloumi is a delicious and refreshing dish that combines the flavours of a traditional Greek salad with the unique taste and texture of grilled halloumi cheese. Here's a recipe to guide you through the preparation:

Ingredients:

- 1 block of halloumi cheese

- 4-5 tomatoes, chopped

- 1 cucumber, diced; 1 red onion, thinly sliced; 1 green bell pepper, diced

- 1/2 cup Kalamata olives

- 1/2 cup crumbled feta cheese

- 2 tablespoons extra virgin olive oil

- 1 tablespoon of red wine vinegar

- 1 teaspoon dried oregano

- Salt and pepper to taste. Freshly chopped parsley (for garnish)

Instructions:

Preheat your grill or grill pan over
medium-high heat.

Slice the halloumi cheese into 1/2-inch-thick
slices.

Brush each slice of halloumi with olive oil on
both sides.

Grill the halloumi slices for about 2–3
minutes on each side until they have nice
grill marks and are slightly softened.

Remove the grilled halloumi from the grill
and set it aside to cool slightly.

In a large bowl, combine the chopped tomatoes, diced cucumber, sliced red onion, diced bell pepper, and Kalamata olives.

In a small bowl, whisk together the extra virgin olive oil, red wine vinegar, dried oregano, salt, and pepper.

Pour the dressing over the salad and toss gently to combine.

Divide the salad into serving plates or bowls.

Place a few slices of grilled halloumi on top of each portion.

Sprinkle crumbled feta cheese over the salad.

Mediterranean Quinoa Salad

Ingredients:

- 1 cup quinoa

- 2 cups water

- 1 cup cherry tomatoes, halved

- 1 cucumber, diced

- 1 red bell pepper, diced

- 1/2 red onion, thinly sliced

- 1/2 cup Kalamata olives, pitted and halved

- 1/2 cup crumbled feta cheese

- 1/4 cup fresh parsley, chopped

- 1/4 cup fresh mint, chopped

For the dressing:

- 1/4 cup extra-virgin olive oil

- 2 tablespoons lemon juice

- 2 cloves garlic, minced

- 1 teaspoon dried oregano

- Salt and pepper to taste

Instructions:

Rinse the quinoa under cold water to remove any bitterness. In a saucepan, combine the quinoa and water. Bring to a boil, then reduce the heat to low and cover. Simmer for about 15 minutes or until the quinoa is tender and the water is absorbed. Remove from heat and let it cool.

In a large bowl, combine the cooked quinoa, cherry tomatoes, cucumber, red bell pepper, red onion, Kalamata olives, feta cheese, parsley, and mint. Toss gently to mix everything together.

In a small bowl, whisk together the olive oil, lemon juice, minced garlic, dried oregano, salt, and pepper. Pour the dressing over the quinoa salad and toss to coat all the ingredients evenly.

Let the salad sit for about 15 minutes to allow the flavours to meld together. You can serve it immediately or refrigerate it for later use.

This Mediterranean Quinoa Salad is packed with fresh vegetables, herbs, and tangy flavours. It makes a delicious and nutritious side dish or a light meal on its own. Enjoy!

Tuscan Panzanella salad

Tuscan Panzanella Salad is a traditional Italian salad hailing from the region of Tuscany. It is a refreshing and vibrant dish that makes use of stale bread, tomatoes, cucumbers, onions, and fresh basil. The salad is dressed with a simple vinaigrette made with olive oil, vinegar, garlic, and salt. Here's a basic recipe to help you make a delicious Tuscan panzanella salad:

Ingredients:

- 4 cups stale bread, torn into bite-sized pieces

- 2 cups ripe tomatoes, chopped

- 1 cucumber, peeled, seeded, and sliced

- 1/2 red onion, thinly sliced

- 1/2 cup fresh basil leaves, torn

- 3 tablespoons of extra-virgin olive oil

- 1 tablespoon of red wine vinegar

- 1 clove of garlic, minced

- Salt and pepper to taste

Instructions:

In a large bowl, combine the torn bread, tomatoes, cucumber slices, red onion, and torn basil leaves.

In a separate small bowl, whisk together the olive oil, red wine vinegar, minced garlic, salt, and pepper to make the vinaigrette.

Pour the vinaigrette over the bread and vegetable mixture, tossing gently to coat everything evenly.

Allow the salad to sit for about 10–15 minutes to allow the flavours to meld together and the bread to soak up the dressing. Toss occasionally during this time.

Before serving, taste and adjust the seasonings if needed, adding more salt, pepper, or vinegar according to your preference.

Serve the Tuscan Panzanella Salad at room temperature and enjoy!

Feel free to customise your panzanella salad by adding other ingredients like bell peppers, olives, or even some mozzarella cheese. It's a versatile salad that can be adapted to suit your taste.

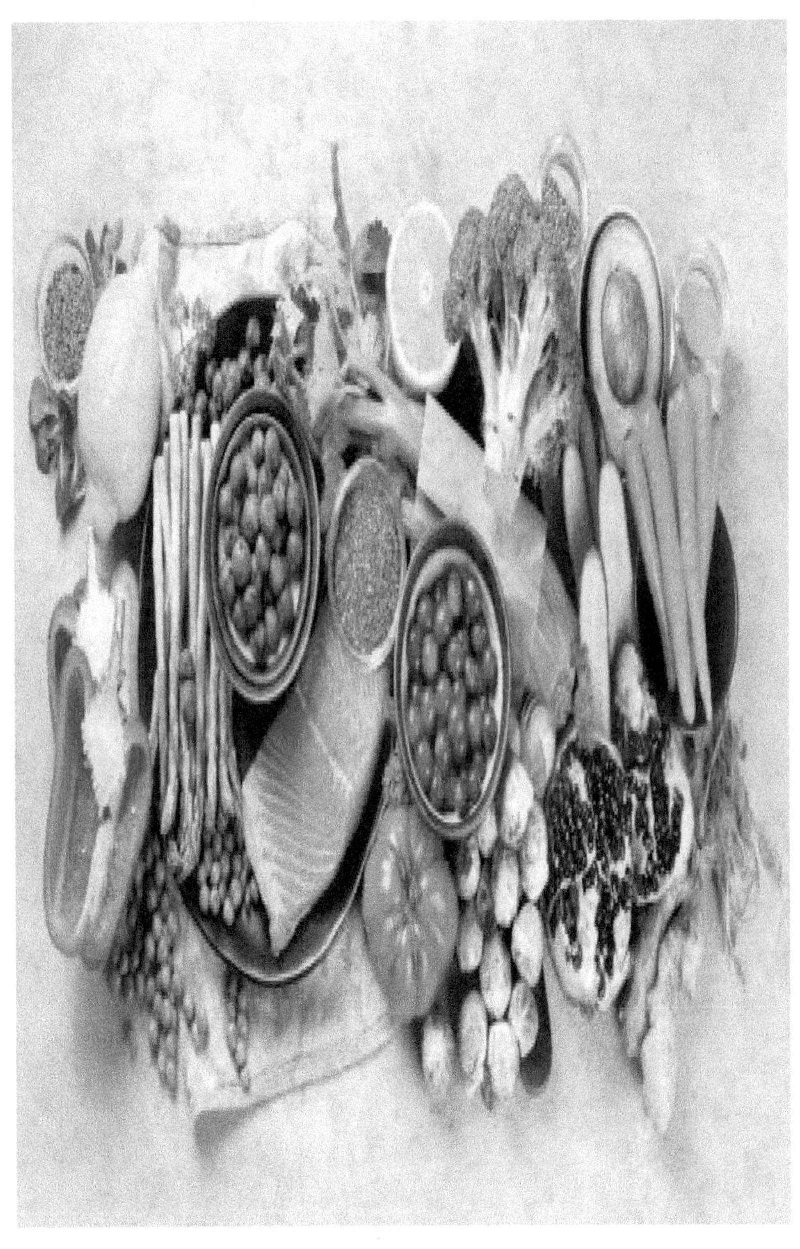

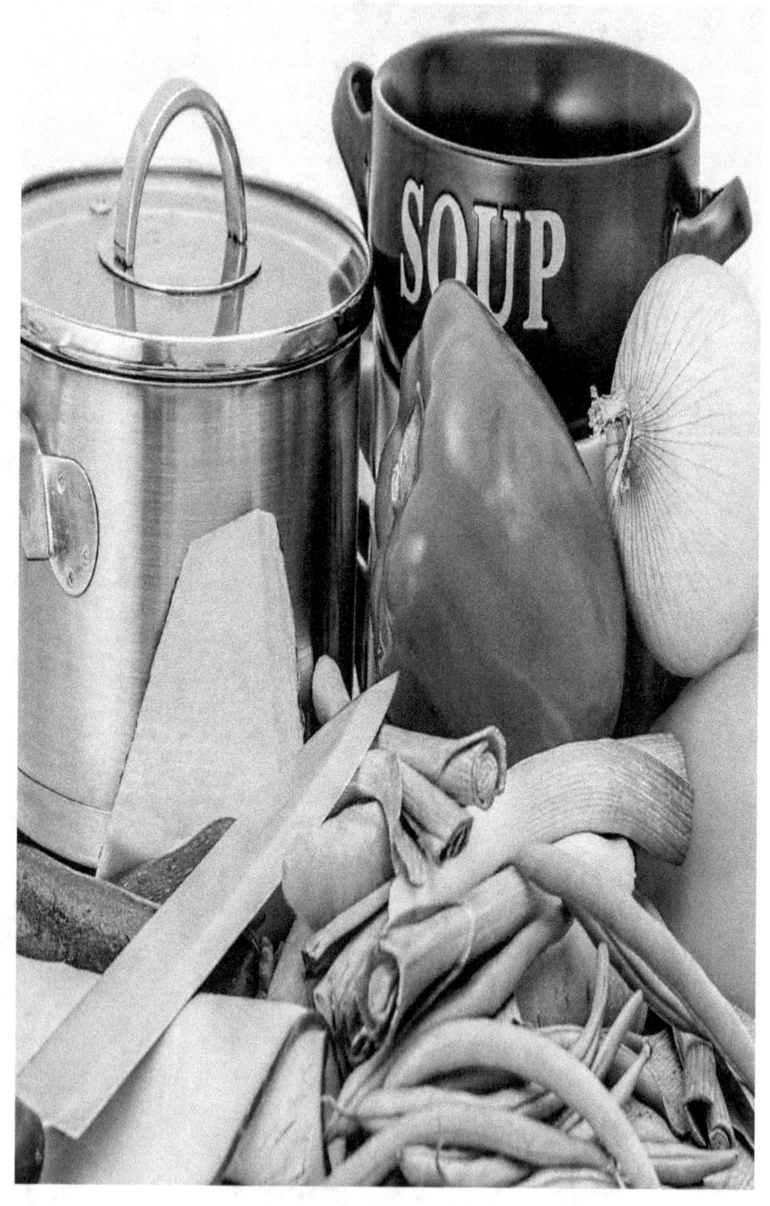
SOUP

Conclusion: Embracing the Mediterranean lifestyle

embracing the Mediterranean lifestyle is a wise choice for individuals seeking a balanced and healthy way of living. Lifestyle, inspired by the eating habits and cultural practices of countries bordering the Mediterranean Sea, offers a wealth of benefits for both physical and mental well-being.

One of the key pillars of the Mediterranean lifestyle is a focus on fresh, whole foods. The emphasis on fruits, vegetables, legumes, whole grains, and lean proteins provide well-being. t-rich diet that is associated with reduced risks of chronic diseases, including heart disease, diabetes, and certain types of cancer. Moreover, the moderate consumption of fish, olive oil, and nuts provides essential omega-3 fatty acids and other beneficial nutrients that promote brain health and overall vitality.

The Mediterranean lifestyle also encourages an active lifestyle. Regular physical activity, such as walking, swimming, or practising yoga, is an integral part of daily route vitality. Mediterranean cultures. This active approach not only helps maintain a healthy weight but also boosts cardiovascular health, improves mood, and enhances overall fitness.

Furthermore, the Mediterranean lifestyle places great importance on social connections and community engagement. The tradition of gathering with friends and family for shared meals fosters a sense of belonging, strengthens relationships, and promotes mental well-being. This communal aspect of the Mediterranean lifestyle can help combat feelings of isolation and loneliness, which have become increasingly prevalent in modern society.

In addition to its positive impact on physical health and social well-being, the Mediterranean lifestyle encourages a more mindful and balanced approach to life. The enjoyment of meals, savouring the flavours and textures of food, and being present in the moment during shared experiences all contribute to a greater sense of fulfilment.

This mindset of mindfulness extends beyond the dinner table, encouraging individuals to prioritise self-care, stress management, and work-life balance.

By embracing the Mediterranean lifestyle, individuals can reap the rewards of improved health, increased vitality, and enhanced overall well-being. While adopting this lifestyle may require adjustments and changes in habits, the long-term benefits far outweigh the initial effort. Embracing the Mediterranean lifestyle is an investment in one's health and happiness, and it offers a pathway to a more fulfilling and vibrant life.

Additional resources for the Mediterranean diet

The Mediterranean Diet is known for its health benefits and emphasis on whole foods, fresh produce, lean proteins, and healthy fats. Here are some additional resources that can provide you with more information, recipes, and guidance on following the Mediterranean Diet:

"The Mediterranean Diet for Beginners:

The Complete Guide: 40 Delicious Recipes, a 7-Day Diet Meal Plan, and 10 Tips for Success"

This book offers a comprehensive guide to getting started with the Mediterranean Diet, including an introduction to the diet's principles, a 7-day meal plan, and a variety of delicious recipes.

Oldways Mediterranean Diet

Oldways is a non-profit organisation that promotes traditional and healthy eating patterns, including the Mediterranean Diet. They provide a wealth of resources on their website, including recipes, meal plans, shopping guides, and cooking tips.

The Mediterranean Dish is a popular website that focuses on Mediterranean cuisine. It offers a wide range of recipes inspired by the Mediterranean Diet, along with cooking tips, ingredient guides, and informative articles.

American Heart Association

The American Heart Association provides information and resources on various heart-healthy diets, including the Mediterranean Diet. Their website offers recipes, meal planning tips, and guidance on adopting a Mediterranean-style eating pattern.

Mayo Clinic:

The Mayo Clinic website features a section dedicated to the Mediterranean Diet, providing an overview of its health benefits, food recommendations, and sample meal plans. They also offer recipes and cooking tips to help you incorporate Mediterranean flavours into your meals.

The Mediterranean Diet Cookbook: 500 Simple Recipes for Beginners and Advanced Users by Emily Wagner

This cookbook offers a wide selection of Mediterranean-inspired recipes suitable for both beginners and those more familiar with the diet. It includes simple and easy-to-follow instructions, making it a useful resource for anyone looking to incorporate the Mediterranean Diet into their lifestyle.

Remember to consult with a healthcare professional or registered dietitian before making any significant changes to your diet, especially if you have specific health concerns or dietary restrictions. These additional resources should help you explore and enjoy the Mediterranean Diet to its fullest.

Tips for successful meal planning

Planning is a great way to save time, money, and effort in your daily life. Here are some tips for successful meal planning:

Set a schedule. Determine how often you want to plan your meals, whether it's weekly, biweekly, or monthly. Having a schedule will help you stay organised and ensure you always have a plan in place.

Consider your lifestyle and preferences. Take into account your dietary needs, personal preferences, and any specific goals you have, such as weight loss or building muscle. Plan meals that align with these factors to make sure you enjoy what you eat.

Take inventory: Before you start planning your meals, check your pantry, refrigerator, and freezer to see what ingredients you already have. This will help you avoid buying unnecessary items and reduce food waste.

Plan balanced meals. Aim for a balance of macronutrients (carbohydrates, proteins, and fats) and include a variety of fruits, vegetables, whole grains, and lean proteins in your meals. This will ensure you're getting a well-rounded diet.

Use a meal planning template: Consider using a meal planning template or app to help you organise your meals. This can make the process easier and allow you to see your plan at a glance.

Plan for leftovers: Cooking larger portions and planning for leftovers can save you time and effort. Designate specific days for leftovers or repurpose them into new dishes to avoid food waste.

Prep in advance: Take some time each week to prep ingredients in advance, such as chopping vegetables or marinating meat. This can save you time during busy weekdays and make cooking feel more manageable.

Create a shopping list. Once you've planned your meals, create a shopping list based on the ingredients you need. Stick to your list when you go grocery shopping to avoid impulse purchases.

Shop with seasonal produce: Opt for seasonal fruits and vegetables, as they are often fresher and more affordable. They can also add variety to your meals throughout the year.

Glossary for Mediterranean ingredients

ingredients:

Olive Oil: A staple in Mediterranean cuisine, olive oil is used for cooking, dressing salads, and adding flavour to various dishes.

Garlic: Used in many Mediterranean recipes, garlic adds a distinct and pungent flavour to dishes.

Lemon: Lemons are frequently used in Mediterranean cooking to add acidity and brightness to dishes. Lemon juice and zest are commonly used.

Tomatoes: Tomatoes are widely used in Mediterranean cuisine, whether fresh or in the form of canned tomato sauce, paste, or diced tomatoes.

Feta Cheese: A popular Mediterranean cheese made from sheep's or goat's milk It has a tangy and salty flavour and is often crumbled over salads or used in various dishes.

Olives: Mediterranean cuisine features a wide variety of olives, which are often used as a snack, in salads, or as a flavouring agent in various dishes.

Capers: These small, pickled flower buds are commonly used in Mediterranean cooking to add a tangy and salty flavour to dishes like pasta, fish, and salads.

Basil is a fragrant herb commonly used in Mediterranean cuisine, especially in Italian dishes like pesto.

Oregano: Another popular herb in Mediterranean cooking, oregano is used to add flavour to many dishes, including pizzas, pasta sauces, and roasted vegetables.

Chickpeas: A versatile legume commonly used in Mediterranean cuisine, chickpeas are used in dishes like hummus, falafel, and stews.

Couscous: A North African staple, couscous is made from crushed durum wheat semolina and is used as a base for many Mediterranean dishes.

Tahini: A paste made from ground sesame seeds, tahini is a key ingredient in Middle Eastern dishes like hummus and tahini sauce.

Za'atar is a Middle Eastern spice blend consisting of thyme, sumac, sesame seeds, and salt. It is commonly used as a seasoning for bread, meat, and vegetables.

Pomegranate: Pomegranate seeds or juice are used in Mediterranean cuisine to add a sweet and tart flavour to salads, sauces, and desserts.

Pine Nuts: These small, creamy nuts are commonly used in Mediterranean dishes like pesto, salads, and desserts.

Eggplant is a versatile vegetable used in various Mediterranean dishes, such as moussaka, ratatouille, and baba ganoush.

Artichokes: Artichokes are often used in Mediterranean cooking, both fresh and preserved, and are enjoyed in dishes like salads, stews, and pasta.

Caperberries: Larger than capers, caperberries are the fruit of the caper bush and are commonly used as a garnish in Mediterranean dishes.

Anchovies: small, oily fish commonly used as a flavouring agent in Mediterranean dishes such as pasta sauces, salads, and pizza.

Saffron: A highly prized spice derived from the crocus flower, saffron adds a unique and aromatic flavour to Mediterranean dishes such as paella and risotto.

This glossary provides a starting point for exploring Mediterranean ingredients, but the cuisine is diverse and varies across different regions.